Happy + Healthy 2021 Planner

Welcome to your new best friend,
the Happy + Healthy 2021 life planner.

I created this planner as a tool to help you take control of your
life, both in your daily tasks and your long term routines.
Wellness-specific features like the daily workout planner,
the monthly habit tracker and the weekly meal sections will help
you build healthier habits & hit your 2021 goals. I firmly believe
that just hoping for the life you want is not enough – it takes
routines, healthy decisions, reminders and clear intentions to
get you to the Happy + Healthy life you're craving.

Let's do it together!

Cheers to your best year yet,

Olivia

(@skinnyhangover)

Important Dates

JANUARY

FEBRUARY

MARCH

APRIL

MAY

JUNE

JULY

AUGUST

SEPTEMBER

OCTOBER

NOVEMBER

DECEMBER

January 2021

SUNDAY	MONDAY	TUESD
3	4	
10	11	
17	18	
24	25	
31		

NESDAY	THURSDAY	FRIDAY	SATURDAY
		1	2
6	7	8	9
13	14	15	16
20	21	22	23
27	28	29	30

January 2021

AT A GLANCE

January Goals:

....

....

....

January Birthdays:

....

....

....

January Anniversaries:

....

....

....

January To Do:

☐ ....

☐ ....

☐ ....

☐ ....

☐ ....

☐ ....

☐ ....

☐ ....

☐ ....

Habit Tracker

Habit	1	2	3	4	5	6	7	8	9	10	11	1.

GRATITUDE:

....
....
....

SHOPPING LIST:

....
....
....
....
....
....
....
....
....
....

BUDGET:

....
....
....

Notes:

....
....
....

5	16	17	18	19	20	21	22	23	24	25	26	27	28	29	30	31

January 2021

MONDAY, 28

- ....
- ....
- ....
- ....

WORKOUT:

....

....

....

TUESDAY, 29

- ....
- ....
- ....
- ....

WORKOUT:

....

....

....

WEDNESDAY, 30

- ....
- ....
- ....
- ....

WORKOUT:

....

....

....

THURSDAY, 31

- ....
- ....
- ....
- ....

WORKOUT:

....

....

....

HAPPY + HEALTHY INTENTION:

....

WORKOUT:
....
....
....
....

FRIDAY, 1

WORKOUT:
....
....
....

SATURDAY, 2

WORKOUT:
....
....
....

SUNDAY, 3

Weekly Eats:

....
....
....
....
....

To Do:

....
....
....
....
....

January 2021

MONDAY, 4

WORKOUT:

- ....
- ....
- ....
- ....

TUESDAY, 5

WORKOUT:

- ....
- ....
- ....
- ....

WEDNESDAY, 6

WORKOUT:

- ....
- ....
- ....
- ....

THURSDAY, 7

WORKOUT:

- ....
- ....
- ....
- ....

HAPPY + HEALTHY INTENTION:

....

WORKOUT:

....

....

....

....

FRIDAY, 8

WORKOUT:

....

....

....

SATURDAY, 9

WORKOUT:

....

....

....

SUNDAY, 10

Weekly Eats:

....

....

....

....

To Do:

....

....

....

....

....

January 2021

MONDAY, 11

-
-
-
-

WORKOUT:

TUESDAY, 12

-
-
-
-

WORKOUT:

WEDNESDAY, 13

-
-
-
-

WORKOUT:

THURSDAY, 14

-
-
-
-

WORKOUT:

HAPPY + HEALTHY INTENTION:

....

WORKOUT:

....

....

....

....

FRIDAY, 15

....

....

....

....

WORKOUT:

....

....

....

SATURDAY, 16

....

....

....

WORKOUT:

....

....

....

SUNDAY, 17

....

....

....

Weekly Eats:

....

....

....

....

....

To Do:

....

....

....

....

....

January 2021

MONDAY, 18

- ....
- ....
- ....
- ....

WORKOUT:
....
....
....
....

TUESDAY, 19

- ....
- ....
- ....
- ....

WORKOUT:
....
....
....
....

WEDNESDAY, 20

- ....
- ....
- ....
- ....

WORKOUT:
....
....
....
....

THURSDAY, 21

- ....
- ....
- ....
- ....

WORKOUT:
....
....
....

....

WORKOUT:

....

....

....

....

FRIDAY, 22

WORKOUT:

....

....

....

SATURDAY, 23

WORKOUT:

....

....

....

SUNDAY, 24

Weekly Eats:

....

....

....

....

....

To Do:

....

....

....

....

....

January 2021

MONDAY, 25

- ....
- ....
- ....
- ....

WORKOUT:

....
....
....
....

TUESDAY, 26

- ....
- ....
- ....
- ....

WORKOUT:

....
....
....
....

WEDNESDAY, 27

- ....
- ....
- ....
- ....

WORKOUT:

....
....
....
....

THURSDAY, 28

- ....
- ....
- ....
- ....

WORKOUT:

....
....
....
....

....

WORKOUT:

....

....

....

....

FRIDAY, 29

....

....

....

....

WORKOUT:

....

....

....

SATURDAY, 30

....

....

....

WORKOUT:

....

....

....

SUNDAY, 31

....

....

....

Weekly Eats:

....

....

....

....

To Do:

....

....

....

....

....

SUNDAY	MONDAY	TUESD
	1	
7	8	
14	15	
21	22	
28		

February 2021

WEDNESDAY	THURSDAY	FRIDAY	SATURDAY
3	4	5	6
10	11	12	13
17	18	19	20
24	25	26	27

February 2021

February Goals:

....
....
....

February Birthdays:

....
....
....

February Anniversaries:

....
....
....

February To Do:

☐ ....

☐ ....

☐ ....

☐ ....

☐ ....

☐ ....

☐ ....

☐ ....

☐ ....

Habit Tracker

Habit	1	2	3	4	5	6	7	8	9

GRATITUDE:

SHOPPING LIST:

BUDGET:

Notes:

13	14	15	16	17	18	19	20	21	22	23	24	25	26	27	28

February 2021

MONDAY, 1

- ....
- ....
- ....
- ....

WORKOUT:

....

....

....

TUESDAY, 2

- ....
- ....
- ....
- ....

WORKOUT:

....

....

....

WEDNESDAY, 3

- ....
- ....
- ....
- ....

WORKOUT:

....

....

....

THURSDAY, 4

- ....
- ....
- ....
- ....

WORKOUT:

....

....

....

....

WORKOUT:

....

....

....

FRIDAY, 5

WORKOUT:

....

....

....

SATURDAY, 6

WORKOUT:

....

....

....

SUNDAY, 7

Weekly Eats:

....

....

....

....

....

To Do:

....

....

....

....

....

February 2021

MONDAY, 8

- ....
- ....
- ....
- ....

WORKOUT:

....
....
....
....

TUESDAY, 9

- ....
- ....
- ....
- ....

WORKOUT:

....
....
....
....

WEDNESDAY, 10

- ....
- ....
- ....
- ....

WORKOUT:

....
....
....
....

THURSDAY, 11

- ....
- ....
- ....
- ....

WORKOUT:

....
....
....
....

....

WORKOUT:

....
....
....
....

FRIDAY, 12

....

WORKOUT:

....
....
....

SATURDAY, 13

....

WORKOUT:

....
....
....

SUNDAY, 14

Weekly Eats:

....
....
....
....
....

To Do:

....
....
....
....
....

February 2021

MONDAY, 15

- ....
- ....
- ....
- ....

WORKOUT:
....
....
....

TUESDAY, 16

- ....
- ....
- ....
- ....

WORKOUT:
....
....
....

WEDNESDAY, 17

- ....
- ....
- ....
- ....

WORKOUT:
....
....
....

THURSDAY, 18

- ....
- ....
- ....
- ....

WORKOUT:
....
....
....

....

	WORKOUT:	FRIDAY, 19
....	....	
....	....	
....	....	
....		

	WORKOUT:	SATURDAY, 20
....	....	
....	....	
....	....	

	WORKOUT:	SUNDAY, 21
....	....	
....	....	
....	....	

Weekly Eats:

....

....

....

....

....

To Do

....

....

....

....

....

February 2021

MONDAY, 22

- ....
- ....
- ....
- ....

WORKOUT:

....
....
....
....

TUESDAY, 23

- ....
- ....
- ....
- ....

WORKOUT:

....
....
....
....

WEDNESDAY, 24

- ....
- ....
- ....
- ....

WORKOUT:

....
....
....
....

THURSDAY, 25

- ....
- ....
- ....
- ....

WORKOUT:

....
....
....

....

WORKOUT:

....

....

....

....

FRIDAY, 26

WORKOUT:

....

....

....

SATURDAY, 27

WORKOUT:

....

....

....

SUNDAY, 28

Weekly Eats:

....

....

....

....

To Do:

....

....

....

....

....

March 2021

SUNDAY	MONDAY	TUESD
	1	
7	8	
14	15	
21	22	
28	29	

WEDNESDAY	THURSDAY	FRIDAY	SATURDAY
3	4	5	6
10	11	12	13
17	18	19	20
24	25	26	27
31			

March 2021

AT A GLANCE

March Goals:

....

....

....

March Birthdays:

....

....

....

March Anniversaries:

....

....

....

March To Do:

☐ ....

☐ ....

☐ ....

☐ ....

☐ ....

☐ ....

☐ ....

☐ ....

☐ ....

Habit Tracker

Habit	1	2	3	4	5	6	7	8	9	10	11	12

GRATITUDE:

SHOPPING LIST:

BUDGET:

Notes:

	16	17	18	19	20	21	22	23	24	25	26	27	28	29	30	31

March 2021

MONDAY, 1

- ....
- ....
- ....
- ....

WORKOUT:

....

....

....

....

TUESDAY, 2

- ....
- ....
- ....
- ....

WORKOUT:

....

....

....

....

WEDNESDAY, 3

- ....
- ....
- ....
- ....

WORKOUT:

....

....

....

....

THURSDAY, 4

- ....
- ....
- ....
- ....

WORKOUT:

....

....

....

....

HAPPY + HEALTHY INTENTION:

....

WORKOUT:

....

....

....

....

FRIDAY, 5

WORKOUT:

....

....

....

SATURDAY, 6

WORKOUT:

....

....

....

SUNDAY, 7

Weekly Eats:

....

....

....

....

....

To Do:

....

....

....

....

March 2021

MONDAY, 8

- ....
- ....
- ....
- ....

WORKOUT:

....
....
....
....

TUESDAY, 9

- ....
- ....
- ....
- ....

WORKOUT:

....
....
....
....

WEDNESDAY, 10

- ....
- ....
- ....
- ....

WORKOUT:

....
....
....
....

THURSDAY, 11

- ....
- ....
- ....
- ....

WORKOUT:

....
....
....
....

HAPPY + HEALTHY INTENTION:

....

WORKOUT:

....
....
....
....

FRIDAY, 12

WORKOUT:

....
....
....

SATURDAY, 13

WORKOUT:

....
....
....

SUNDAY, 14

Weekly Eats

....

....

....

....

To Do

....

....

....

....

....

March 2021

MONDAY, 15

- ....
- ....
- ....
- ....

WORKOUT:

....
....
....
....

TUESDAY, 16

- ....
- ....
- ....
- ....

WORKOUT:

....
....
....
....

WEDNESDAY, 17

- ....
- ....
- ....
- ....

WORKOUT:

....
....
....
....

THURSDAY, 18

- ....
- ....
- ....
- ....

WORKOUT:

....
....
....
....

HAPPY + HEALTHY INTENTION:

....

WORKOUT:

....

....

....

....

FRIDAY, 19

WORKOUT:

....

....

....

SATURDAY, 20

WORKOUT:

....

....

....

SUNDAY, 21

Weekly Eats:

....

....

....

....

....

To Do:

....

....

....

....

....

March 2021

MONDAY, 22

-
-
-
-

WORKOUT:

TUESDAY, 23

-
-
-
-

WORKOUT:

WEDNESDAY, 24

-
-
-
-

WORKOUT:

THURSDAY, 25

-
-
-
-

WORKOUT:

HAPPY + HEALTHY INTENTION:

....

FRIDAY, 26

WORKOUT:

....

....

....

....

SATURDAY, 27

WORKOUT:

....

....

....

SUNDAY, 28

WORKOUT:

....

....

....

Weekly Eats

....

....

....

....

....

To Do

....

....

....

....

....

March 2021

MONDAY, 29

WORKOUT:

- ....
- ....
- ....
- ....

TUESDAY, 30

WORKOUT:

- ....
- ....
- ....
- ....

WEDNESDAY, 31

WORKOUT:

- ....
- ....
- ....
- ....

THURSDAY, 1

WORKOUT:

- ....
- ....
- ....
- ....

HAPPY + HEALTHY INTENTION:

....

WORKOUT:

....

....

....

....

FRIDAY, 2

WORKOUT:

....

....

....

SATURDAY, 3

WORKOUT:

....

....

....

SUNDAY, 4

Weekly Eats

....

....

....

....

....

To Do:

....

....

....

....

....

April 2021

SUNDAY	MONDAY	TUESD
4	5	
11	12	
18	19	2
25	26	2

NESDAY	THURSDAY	FRIDAY	SATURDAY
	1	2	3
7	8	9	10
14	15	16	17
21	22	23	24
28	29	30	

April 2021

AT A GLANCE

April Goals:

....

....

....

April Birthdays:

....

....

....

April Anniversaries:

....

....

....

April To Do:

- ☐ ....
- ☐ ....
- ☐ ....
- ☐ ....
- ☐ ....
- ☐ ....
- ☐ ....
- ☐ ....
- ☐ ....

Habit Tracker

Habit	1	2	3	4	5	6	7	8	9	10

GRATITUDE:

SHOPPING LIST:

BUDGET:

Notes:

14	15	16	17	18	19	20	21	22	23	24	25	26	27	28	29	30

April 2021

MONDAY, 5

-
-
-
-

WORKOUT:

TUESDAY, 6

-
-
-
-

WORKOUT:

WEDNESDAY, 7

-
-
-
-

WORKOUT:

THURSDAY, 8

-
-
-
-

WORKOUT:

....

WORKOUT:

....

....

....

....

FRIDAY, 9

WORKOUT:

....

....

....

SATURDAY, 10

WORKOUT:

....

....

....

SUNDAY, 11

Weekly Eats

....

....

....

....

....

To Do:

....

....

....

....

....

April 2021

MONDAY, 12

- ....
- ....
- ....
- ....

WORKOUT:

....
....
....
....

TUESDAY, 13

- ....
- ....
- ....
- ....

WORKOUT:

....
....
....
....

WEDNESDAY, 14

- ....
- ....
- ....
- ....

WORKOUT:

....
....
....
....

THURSDAY, 15

- ....
- ....
- ....
- ....

WORKOUT:

....
....
....
....

HAPPY + HEALTHY INTENTION:

....

WORKOUT:

FRIDAY, 16

WORKOUT:

SATURDAY, 17

WORKOUT:

SUNDAY, 18

Weekly Eats:

To Do:

April 2021

MONDAY, 19

- ....
- ....
- ....
- ....

WORKOUT:

....
....
....
....

TUESDAY, 20

- ....
- ....
- ....
- ....

WORKOUT:

....
....
....
....

WEDNESDAY, 21

- ....
- ....
- ....
- ....

WORKOUT:

....
....
....
....

THURSDAY, 22

- ....
- ....
- ....
- ....

WORKOUT:

....
....
....
....

HAPPY + HEALTHY INTENTION:

....

WORKOUT:

....

....

....

....

FRIDAY, 23

WORKOUT:

....

....

....

SATURDAY, 24

WORKOUT:

....

....

....

SUNDAY, 25

Weekly Eats:

....

....

....

....

To Do:

....

....

....

....

April 2021

MONDAY, 26

- ....
- ....
- ....
- ....

WORKOUT:

....
....
....
....

TUESDAY, 27

- ....
- ....
- ....
- ....

WORKOUT:

....
....
....
....

WEDNESDAY, 28

- ....
- ....
- ....
- ....

WORKOUT:

....
....
....
....

THURSDAY, 29

- ....
- ....
- ....
- ....

WORKOUT:

....
....
....
....

....

WORKOUT:

FRIDAY, 30

....

....

....

....

WORKOUT:

SATURDAY, 1

....

....

....

WORKOUT:

SUNDAY, 2

....

....

....

Weekly Eats

....

....

....

....

....

To Do

....

....

....

....

....

May 2021

SUNDAY	MONDAY	TUESD
2	3	
9	10	
16	17	
23	24	
30	31	

NESDAY	THURSDAY	FRIDAY	SATURDAY
			1
5	6	7	8
12	13	14	15
19	20	21	22
26	27	28	29

May 2021

AT A GLANCE

May Goals:

....
....
....

May Birthdays:

....
....
....

May Anniversaries:

....
....
....

May To Do:

- ☐ ....
- ☐ ....
- ☐ ....
- ☐ ....
- ☐ ....
     ....
- ☐ ....
     ....
- ☐ ....
     ....
- ☐ ....
     ....
- ☐ ....

Habit Tracker

Habit	1	2	3	4	5	6	7	8	9	10	11

GRATITUDE:

SHOPPING LIST:

BUDGET:

Notes:

5	16	17	18	19	20	21	22	23	24	25	26	27	28	29	30	31

May 2021

MONDAY, 3

-
-
-
-

WORKOUT:

TUESDAY, 4

-
-
-
-

WORKOUT:

WEDNESDAY, 5

-
-
-
-

WORKOUT:

THURSDAY, 6

-
-
-
-

WORKOUT:

HAPPY + HEALTHY INTENTION:

WORKOUT:

FRIDAY, 7

WORKOUT:

SATURDAY, 8

WORKOUT:

SUNDAY, 9

Weekly Eats:

To Do

May 2021

MONDAY, 10

-
-
-
-

WORKOUT:

TUESDAY, 11

-
-
-
-

WORKOUT:

WEDNESDAY, 12

-
-
-
-

WORKOUT:

THURSDAY, 13

-
-
-
-

WORKOUT:

....

WORKOUT:

....

....

....

....

....

FRIDAY, 14

WORKOUT:

....

....

....

SATURDAY, 15

WORKOUT:

....

....

....

SUNDAY, 16

Weekly Eats:

To Do:

....

....

....

....

....

....

....

....

....

....

May 2021

MONDAY, 17

-
-
-
-

WORKOUT:

TUESDAY, 18

-
-
-
-

WORKOUT:

WEDNESDAY, 19

-
-
-
-

WORKOUT:

THURSDAY, 20

-
-
-
-

WORKOUT:

HAPPY + HEALTHY INTENTION:

WORKOUT:

FRIDAY, 21

WORKOUT:

SATURDAY, 22

WORKOUT:

SUNDAY, 23

Weekly Eats:

To Do:

May 2021

MONDAY, 24

-
-
-
-

WORKOUT:

TUESDAY, 25

-
-
-
-

WORKOUT:

WEDNESDAY, 26

-
-
-
-

WORKOUT:

THURSDAY, 27

-
-
-
-

WORKOUT:

....

WORKOUT:

....
....
....
....

FRIDAY, 28

....

....

....

WORKOUT:

....
....
....

SATURDAY, 29

....

....

....

WORKOUT:

....
....
....

SUNDAY, 30

Weekly Eats:

....
....
....
....
....

To Do:

....
....
....
....
....

June 2021

SUNDAY	MONDAY	TUESD
6	7	
13	14	
20	21	
27	28	

NESDAY	THURSDAY	FRIDAY	SATURDAY
2	3	4	5
9	10	11	12
16	17	18	19
23	24	25	26
30			

June 2021

AT A GLANCE

June Goals:

....
....
....

June Birthdays:

....
....
....

June Anniversaries:

....
....
....

June To Do:

- ☐ ....
- ☐ ....
- ☐ ....
- ☐ ....
- ☐ ....
- ☐ ....
- ☐ ....
- ☐ ....
- ☐ ....

Habit Tracker

Habit	1	2	3	4	5	6	7	8	9	10	

GRATITUDE:

SHOPPING LIST:

BUDGET:

Notes:

14	15	16	17	18	19	20	21	22	23	24	25	26	27	28	29	30

June 2021

MONDAY, 31

-
-
-
-

WORKOUT:

TUESDAY, 1

-
-
-
-

WORKOUT:

WEDNESDAY, 2

-
-
-
-

WORKOUT:

THURSDAY, 3

-
-
-
-

WORKOUT:

HAPPY + HEALTHY INTENTION:

....

WORKOUT:

....

....

....

....

FRIDAY, 4

WORKOUT:

....

....

....

SATURDAY, 5

WORKOUT:

....

....

....

SUNDAY, 6

Weekly Eats

To Do

June 2021

MONDAY, 7

- ....
- ....
- ....
- ....

WORKOUT:

....

....

....

TUESDAY, 8

- ....
- ....
- ....
- ....

WORKOUT:

....

....

....

WEDNESDAY, 9

- ....
- ....
- ....
- ....

WORKOUT:

....

....

....

THURSDAY, 10

- ....
- ....
- ....
- ....

WORKOUT:

....

....

....

HAPPY + HEALTHY INTENTION:

....

WORKOUT:

....

....

....

....

FRIDAY, 11

....

....

....

WORKOUT:

....

....

....

SATURDAY, 12

....

....

....

WORKOUT:

....

....

....

SUNDAY, 13

Weekly Eats:

....

....

....

....

....

To Do:

....

....

....

....

....

June 2021

MONDAY, 14

- ....
- ....
- ....
- ....

WORKOUT:

TUESDAY, 15

- ....
- ....
- ....
- ....

WORKOUT:

WEDNESDAY, 16

- ....
- ....
- ....
- ....

WORKOUT:

THURSDAY, 17

- ....
- ....
- ....
- ....

WORKOUT:

....

WORKOUT:

....

....

....

....

FRIDAY, 18

WORKOUT:

....

....

....

SATURDAY, 19

WORKOUT:

....

....

....

SUNDAY, 20

Weekly Eats:

....

....

....

....

....

To Do:

....

....

....

....

....

June 2021

MONDAY, 21

- ....
- ....
- ....
- ....

WORKOUT:
....
....
....
....

TUESDAY, 22

- ....
- ....
- ....
- ....

WORKOUT:
....
....
....
....

WEDNESDAY, 23

- ....
- ....
- ....
- ....

WORKOUT:
....
....
....
....

THURSDAY, 24

- ....
- ....
- ....
- ....

WORKOUT:
....
....
....
....

....

WORKOUT:

....

....

....

....

FRIDAY, 25

WORKOUT:

....

....

....

SATURDAY, 26

WORKOUT:

....

....

....

SUNDAY, 27

Weekly Eats

....

....

....

....

....

To Do:

....

....

....

....

....

June 2021

MONDAY, 28

- ....
- ....
- ....
- ....

WORKOUT:

....
....
....
....

TUESDAY, 29

- ....
- ....
- ....
- ....

WORKOUT:

....
....
....
....

WEDNESDAY, 30

- ....
- ....
- ....
- ....

WORKOUT:

....
....
....
....

THURSDAY, 1

- ....
- ....
- ....
- ....

WORKOUT:

....
....
....
....

HAPPY + HEALTHY INTENTION:

....

WORKOUT:

....

....

....

....

FRIDAY, 2

WORKOUT:

....

....

....

SATURDAY, 3

WORKOUT:

....

....

....

SUNDAY, 4

Weekly Eats

....

....

....

....

To Do

....

....

....

....

....

SUNDAY	MONDAY	TUESD
4	5	
11	12	
18	19	
25	26	

July 2021

WEDNESDAY	THURSDAY	FRIDAY	SATURDAY
	1	2	3
7	8	9	10
14	15	16	17
21	22	23	24
28	29	30	31

July 2021

AT A GLANCE

July Goals:

....

....

....

July Birthdays:

....

....

....

July Anniversaries:

....

....

....

July To Do:

- ☐ ....
- ☐ ....
- ☐ ....
- ☐ ....
- ☐ ....
- ☐ ....
- ☐ ....
- ☐ ....
- ☐ ....

Habit Tracker

Habit	1	2	3	4	5	6	7	8	9	10	11	1

GRATITUDE:

SHOPPING LIST:

BUDGET:

Notes:

5	16	17	18	19	20	21	22	23	24	25	26	27	28	29	30	31

July 2021

MONDAY, 5

- ....
- ....
- ....
- ....

WORKOUT:

....

....

....

....

TUESDAY, 6

- ....
- ....
- ....
- ....

WORKOUT:

....

....

....

....

WEDNESDAY, 7

- ....
- ....
- ....
- ....

WORKOUT:

....

....

....

....

THURSDAY, 8

- ....
- ....
- ....
- ....

WORKOUT:

....

....

....

....

....

	WORKOUT:	FRIDAY, 9
....	....	
....	....	
....	....	
....	....	

	WORKOUT:	SATURDAY, 10
....	....	
....	....	
....	....	

	WORKOUT:	SUNDAY, 11
....	....	
....	....	
....	....	

Weekly Eats:

....

....

....

....

....

To Do

....

....

....

....

....

July 2021

MONDAY, 12

- ....
- ....
- ....
- ....

WORKOUT:

....
....
....
....

TUESDAY, 13

- ....
- ....
- ....
- ....

WORKOUT:

....
....
....
....

WEDNESDAY, 14

- ....
- ....
- ....
- ....

WORKOUT:

....
....
....
....

THURSDAY, 15

- ....
- ....
- ....
- ....

WORKOUT:

....
....
....
....

....

WORKOUT:

....

....

....

....

FRIDAY, 16

WORKOUT:

....

....

....

SATURDAY, 17

WORKOUT:

....

....

....

SUNDAY, 18

Weekly Eats

....

....

....

....

To Do

....

....

....

....

....

July 2021

MONDAY, 19

- ....
- ....
- ....
- ....

WORKOUT:

TUESDAY, 20

- ....
- ....
- ....
- ....

WORKOUT:

WEDNESDAY, 21

- ....
- ....
- ....
- ....

WORKOUT:

THURSDAY, 22

- ....
- ....
- ....
- ....

WORKOUT:

HAPPY + HEALTHY INTENTION:

....

WORKOFF:

FRIDAY, 23

WORKOUT:

SATURDAY, 24

WORKOUT:

SUNDAY, 25

Weekly Eats

To Do

July 2021

MONDAY, 26

- ....
- ....
- ....
- ....

WORKOUT:

....
....
....
....

TUESDAY, 27

- ....
- ....
- ....
- ....

WORKOUT:

....
....
....
....

WEDNESDAY, 28

- ....
- ....
- ....
- ....

WORKOUT:

....
....
....
....

THURSDAY, 29

- ....
- ....
- ....
- ....

WORKOUT:

....
....
....
....

HAPPY + HEALTHY INTENTION:

....

WORKOUT:

FRIDAY, 30

WORKOUT:

SATURDAY, 31

WORKOUT:

SUNDAY, 1

Weekly Eats:

....

....

....

....

....

To Do:

....

....

....

....

....

August 2021

SUNDAY	MONDAY	TUESD
1	2	
8	9	
15	16	
22	23	
29	30	

WEDNESDAY	THURSDAY	FRIDAY	SATURDAY
4	5	6	7
11	12	13	14
18	19	20	21
25	26	27	28

August 2021

AT A GLANCE

August Goals:

....
....
....

August Birthdays:

....
....
....

August Anniversaries:

....
....
....

August To Do:

- ☐ ....
- ☐ ....
- ☐ ....
- ☐ ....
- ☐ ....
- ☐ ....
- ☐ ....
- ☐ ....
- ☐ ....

Habit Tracker

Habit	1	2	3	4	5	6	7	8	9	10	11	12

GRATITUDE:

SHOPPING LIST:

BUDGET:

Notes:

15	16	17	18	19	20	21	22	23	24	25	26	27	28	29	30	31

August 2021

MONDAY, 2

- ....
- ....
- ....
- ....

WORKOUT:

....
....
....
....

TUESDAY, 3

- ....
- ....
- ....
- ....

WORKOUT:

....
....
....
....

WEDNESDAY, 4

- ....
- ....
- ....
- ....

WORKOUT:

....
....
....
....

THURSDAY, 5

- ....
- ....
- ....
- ....

WORKOUT:

....
....
....
....

....

WORKOUT:

....

....

....

....

FRIDAY, 6

WORKOUT:

....

....

....

....

SATURDAY, 7

WORKOUT:

....

....

....

....

SUNDAY, 8

Weekly Eats:

....

....

....

....

....

To Do:

....

....

....

....

....

August 2021

MONDAY, 9

- ....
- ....
- ....
- ....

WORKOUT:

TUESDAY, 10

- ....
- ....
- ....
- ....

WORKOUT:

WEDNESDAY, 11

- ....
- ....
- ....
- ....

WORKOUT:

THURSDAY, 12

- ....
- ....
- ....
- ....

WORKOUT:

....

WORKOUT:

....

....

....

....

FRIDAY, 13

WORKOUT:

....

....

....

SATURDAY, 14

WORKOUT:

....

....

....

SUNDAY, 15

Weekly Eats:

....

....

....

....

....

To Do:

....

....

....

....

....

August 2021

MONDAY, 16

- ....
- ....
- ....
- ....

WORKOUT:

....

....

....

....

TUESDAY, 17

- ....
- ....
- ....
- ....

WORKOUT:

....

....

....

....

WEDNESDAY, 18

- ....
- ....
- ....
- ....

WORKOUT:

....

....

....

....

THURSDAY, 19

- ....
- ....
- ....
- ....

WORKOUT:

....

....

....

....

HAPPY + HEALTHY INTENTION:

....

FRIDAY, 20

WORKOUT:

....

....

....

....

....

....

....

SATURDAY, 21

WORKOUT:

....

....

....

....

....

....

SUNDAY, 22

WORKOUT:

....

....

....

....

....

....

Weekly Eats:

....

....

....

....

To Do:

....

....

....

....

....

August 2021

MONDAY, 23

- ....
- ....
- ....
- ....

WORKOUT:

....

....

....

....

TUESDAY, 24

- ....
- ....
- ....
- ....

WORKOUT:

....

....

....

....

WEDNESDAY, 25

- ....
- ....
- ....
- ....

WORKOUT:

....

....

....

....

THURSDAY, 26

- ....
- ....
- ....
- ....

WORKOUT:

....

....

....

....

....

WORKOUT:

....

....

....

FRIDAY, 27

....

WORKOUT:

....

....

....

SATURDAY, 28

WORKOUT:

....

....

....

SUNDAY, 29

Weekly Eats:

....

....

....

....

....

To Do:

....

....

....

....

....

September 2021

SUNDAY	MONDAY	TUES...
5	6	
12	13	
19	20	
26	27	

NESDAY	THURSDAY	FRIDAY	SATURDAY
1	2	3	4
8	9	10	11
15	16	17	18
22	23	24	25
29	30		

September 2021

AT A GLANCE

September Goals:

....
....
....

September Birthdays:

....
....
....

September Anniversaries:

....
....
....

September To Do:

☐ ....
☐ ....
☐ ....
☐ ....
☐ ....
☐ ....
☐ ....
☐ ....
☐ ....

Habit Tracker

Habit	1	2	3	4	5	6	7	8	9	10	1

GRATITUDE:

SHOPPING LIST:

BUDGET:

Notes:

4	15	16	17	18	19	20	21	22	23	24	25	26	27	28	29	30

September 2021

MONDAY, 30

- ....
- ....
- ....
- ....

WORKOUT:

....

....

....

....

TUESDAY, 31

- ....
- ....
- ....
- ....

WORKOUT:

....

....

....

....

WEDNESDAY, 1

- ....
- ....
- ....
- ....

WORKOUT:

....

....

....

....

THURSDAY, 2

- ....
- ....
- ....
- ....

WORKOUT:

....

....

....

....

HAPPY + HEALTHY INTENTION:

....

WORKOUT:

....

....

....

....

FRIDAY, 3

WORKOUT:

....

....

....

SATURDAY, 4

WORKOUT:

....

....

....

SUNDAY, 5

Weekly Eats:

....

....

....

....

....

To Do:

....

....

....

....

....

September 2021

MONDAY, 6

WORKOUT:

- ....
- ....
- ....
- ....

TUESDAY, 7

WORKOUT:

- ....
- ....
- ....
- ....

WEDNESDAY, 8

WORKOUT:

- ....
- ....
- ....
- ....

THURSDAY, 9

WORKOUT:

- ....
- ....
- ....
- ....

HAPPY + HEALTHY INTENTION:

....

WORKOUT:

....

....

....

....

FRIDAY, 10

WORKOUT:

....

....

....

SATURDAY, 11

WORKOUT:

....

....

....

SUNDAY, 12

Weekly Eats:

....

....

....

....

To Do:

....

....

....

....

....

September 2021

MONDAY, 13

- ....
- ....
- ....
- ....

WORKOUT:

....

....

....

....

TUESDAY, 14

- ....
- ....
- ....
- ....

WORKOUT:

....

....

....

....

WEDNESDAY, 15

- ....
- ....
- ....
- ....

WORKOUT:

....

....

....

....

THURSDAY, 16

- ....
- ....
- ....
- ....

WORKOUT:

....

....

....

....

....

WORKOUT:

....

....

....

....

FRIDAY, 17

WORKOUT:

....

....

....

SATURDAY, 18

WORKOUT:

....

....

....

SUNDAY, 19

Weekly Eats:

....

....

....

....

....

To Do:

....

....

....

....

....

September 2021

MONDAY, 20

- ....
- ....
- ....
- ....

WORKOUT:

....

....

....

TUESDAY, 21

- ....
- ....
- ....
- ....

WORKOUT:

....

....

....

WEDNESDAY, 22

- ....
- ....
- ....
- ....

WORKOUT:

....

....

....

THURSDAY, 23

- ....
- ....
- ....
- ....

WORKOUT:

....

....

....

....

	WORKOUT:	FRIDAY, 24
....	....	
....	....	
....	....	
....	....	
....		

	WORKOUT:	SATURDAY, 25
....	....	
....	....	
....	....	
....		

	WORKOUT:	SUNDAY, 26
....	....	
....	....	
....	....	
....		

Weekly Eats:

....

....

....

....

....

To Do:

....

....

....

....

....

September 2021

MONDAY, 27

- ....
- ....
- ....
- ....

WORKOUT:
....
....
....
....

TUESDAY, 28

- ....
- ....
- ....
- ....

WORKOUT:
....
....
....
....

WEDNESDAY, 29

- ....
- ....
- ....
- ....

WORKOUT:
....
....
....
....

THURSDAY, 30

- ....
- ....
- ....
- ....

WORKOUT:
....
....
....
....

....

WORKOUT:

....

....

....

....

FRIDAY, 1

WORKOUT:

....

....

....

SATURDAY, 2

WORKOUT:

....

....

....

SUNDAY, 3

Weekly Eats:

....

....

....

....

To Do:

....

....

....

....

....

October 2021

SUNDAY	MONDAY	TUESD
3	4	
10	11	
17	18	
24	25	
31		

NESDAY	THURSDAY	FRIDAY	SATURDAY
		1	2
6	7	8	9
13	14	15	16
20	21	22	23
27	28	29	30

October 2021

AT A GLANCE

October Goals:

....
....
....

October Birthdays:

....
....
....

October Anniversaries:

....
....
....

October To Do:

- [ ] ....
- [ ] ....
- [ ] ....
- [ ] ....
- [ ] ....
- [ ] ....
- [ ] ....
- [ ] ....
- [ ] ....

Habit Tracker

Habit	1	2	3	4	5	6	7	8	9	10	11	

GRATITUDE:

SHOPPING LIST:

BUDGET:

Notes:

16	17	18	19	20	21	22	23	24	25	26	27	28	29	30	31

October 2021

MONDAY, 4

- ....
- ....
- ....
- ....

WORKOUT:

TUESDAY, 5

- ....
- ....
- ....
- ....

WORKOUT:

WEDNESDAY, 6

- ....
- ....
- ....
- ....

WORKOUT:

THURSDAY, 7

- ....
- ....
- ....
- ....

WORKOUT:

HAPPY + HEALTHY INTENTION:

....

WORKOUT:
....
....
....
....

FRIDAY, 8

WORKOUT:
....
....
....

SATURDAY, 9

WORKOUT:
....
....
....

SUNDAY, 10

Weekly Eats:
....
....
....
....
....

To Do:
....
....
....
....
....

October 2021

MONDAY, 11

- ....
- ....
- ....
- ....

WORKOUT:

....
....
....
....

TUESDAY, 12

- ....
- ....
- ....
- ....

WORKOUT:

....
....
....
....

WEDNESDAY, 13

- ....
- ....
- ....
- ....

WORKOUT:

....
....
....
....

THURSDAY, 14

- ....
- ....
- ....
- ....

WORKOUT:

....
....
....
....

HAPPY + HEALTHY INTENTION:

....

WORKOUT:

....

....

....

....

FRIDAY, 15

WORKOUT:

....

....

....

SATURDAY, 16

WORKOUT:

....

....

....

SUNDAY, 17

Weekly Eats

....

....

....

....

To Do

....

....

....

....

....

October 2021

MONDAY, 18

WORKOUT:

- ....
- ....
- ....
- ....

TUESDAY, 19

WORKOUT:

- ....
- ....
- ....
- ....

WEDNESDAY, 20

WORKOUT:

- ....
- ....
- ....
- ....

THURSDAY, 21

WORKOUT:

- ....
- ....
- ....
- ....

HAPPY + HEALTHY INTENTION:

....

WORKOUT:

....

....

....

FRIDAY, 22

WORKOUT:

....

....

....

SATURDAY, 23

WORKOUT:

....

....

....

SUNDAY, 24

Weekly Eats:

....

....

....

....

....

To Do:

....

....

....

....

....

October 2021

MONDAY, 25

- ....
- ....
- ....
- ....

WORKOUT:

....
....
....
....

TUESDAY, 26

- ....
- ....
- ....
- ....

WORKOUT:

....
....
....
....

WEDNESDAY, 27

- ....
- ....
- ....
- ....

WORKOUT:

....
....
....
....

THURSDAY, 28

- ....
- ....
- ....
- ....

WORKOUT:

....
....
....
....

HAPPY + HEALTHY INTENTION:

....

WORKOUT:

....

FRIDAY, 29

WORKOUT:

....

SATURDAY, 30

WORKOUT:

....

SUNDAY, 31

Weekly Eats:

....

To Do:

....

November 2021

SUNDAY	MONDAY	TUESD
	1	
7	8	
14	15	
21	22	
28	29	

WEDNESDAY	THURSDAY	FRIDAY	SATURDAY
3	4	5	6
10	11	12	13
17	18	19	20
24	25	26	27

November 2021

AT A GLANCE

November Goals:
....
....
....

November Birthdays:
....
....
....

November Anniversaries:
....
....
....

November To Do:
☐ ....
☐ ....
☐ ....
☐ ....
☐ ....
....
☐ ....
....
☐ ....
....
....
☐ ....
....
☐ ....

Habit Tracker

Habit	1	2	3	4	5	6	7	8	9	10	

GRATITUDE:

SHOPPING LIST:

BUDGET:

Notes:

15	16	17	18	19	20	21	22	23	24	25	26	27	28	29	30

November 2021

MONDAY, 1

- ....
- ....
- ....
- ....

WORKOUT:

TUESDAY, 2

- ....
- ....
- ....
- ....

WORKOUT:

WEDNESDAY, 3

- ....
- ....
- ....
- ....

WORKOUT:

THURSDAY, 4

- ....
- ....
- ....
- ....

WORKOUT:

....

WORKOUT:
....

....

....

....

FRIDAY, 5

WORKOUT:
....

....

....

SATURDAY, 6

WORKOUT:
....

....

....

SUNDAY, 7

Weekly Eats:

....

....

....

....

....

To Do:

....

....

....

....

....

November 2021

MONDAY, 8

WORKOUT:

TUESDAY, 9

WORKOUT:

WEDNESDAY, 10

WORKOUT:

THURSDAY, 11

WORKOUT:

HAPPY + HEALTHY INTENTION:

WORKOUT:

FRIDAY, 12

WORKOUT:

SATURDAY, 13

WORKOUT:

SUNDAY, 14

Weekly Eats:

To Do:

November 2021

MONDAY, 15

- ....
- ....
- ....
- ....

WORKOUT:

- ....
- ....
- ....
- ....

TUESDAY, 16

- ....
- ....
- ....
- ....

WORKOUT:

- ....
- ....
- ....
- ....

WEDNESDAY, 17

- ....
- ....
- ....
- ....

WORKOUT:

- ....
- ....
- ....
- ....

THURSDAY, 18

- ....
- ....
- ....
- ....

WORKOUT:

- ....
- ....
- ....
- ....

HAPPY + HEALTHY INTENTION:

....

WORKOUT:

....

....

....

....

FRIDAY, 19

WORKOUT:

....

....

....

SATURDAY, 20

WORKOUT:

....

....

....

SUNDAY, 21

Weekly Eats:

....

....

....

....

....

To Do:

....

....

....

....

....

November 2021

MONDAY, 22

-
-
-
-

WORKOUT:

TUESDAY, 23

-
-
-
-

WORKOUT:

WEDNESDAY, 24

-
-
-
-

WORKOUT:

THURSDAY, 25

-
-
-
-

WORKOUT:

....

WORKOUT:

....

....

....

....

FRIDAY, 26

WORKOUT:

....

....

....

SATURDAY, 27

WORKOUT:

....

....

....

SUNDAY, 28

Weekly Eats:

To Do:

November 2021

MONDAY, 29

- ....
- ....
- ....
- ....

WORKOUT:

....
....
....
....

TUESDAY, 30

- ....
- ....
- ....
- ....

WORKOUT:

....
....
....
....

WEDNESDAY, 1

- ....
- ....
- ....
- ....

WORKOUT:

....
....
....
....

THURSDAY, 2

- ....
- ....
- ....
- ....

WORKOUT:

....
....
....

....

WORKOUT:

....

....

....

FRIDAY, 3

WORKOUT:

....

....

....

SATURDAY, 4

WORKOUT:

....

....

....

SUNDAY, 5

Weekly Eats:

....

....

....

....

To Do:

....

....

....

....

....

December 2021

SUNDAY	MONDAY	TUESD
5	6	
12	13	
19	20	
26	27	2

NESDAY	THURSDAY	FRIDAY	SATURDAY
1	2	3	4
8	9	10	11
15	16	17	18
22	23	24	25
29	30	31	

December 2021

AT A GLANCE

December Goals:

....
....
....

December Birthdays:

....
....
....

December Anniversaries:

....
....
....

December To Do:

- ....
- ....
- ....
- ....
- ....
- ....
- ....
- ....

Habit Tracker

Habit	1	2	3	4	5	6	7	8	9	10	11

GRATITUDE:

SHOPPING LIST:

BUDGET:

Notes:

5	16	17	18	19	20	21	22	23	24	25	26	27	28	29	30	31

December 2021

MONDAY, 6

- ....
- ....
- ....
- ....

WORKOUT:

TUESDAY, 7

- ....
- ....
- ....
- ....

WORKOUT:

WEDNESDAY, 8

- ....
- ....
- ....
- ....

WORKOUT:

THURSDAY, 9

- ....
- ....
- ....
- ....

WORKOUT:

HAPPY + HEALTHY INTENTION:

....

WORKOUT:

....

....

....

....

FRIDAY, 10

WORKOUT:

....

....

....

SATURDAY, 11

WORKOUT:

....

....

....

SUNDAY, 12

Weekly Eats:

....

....

....

....

To Do:

....

....

....

....

....

December 2021

MONDAY, 13

-
-
-
-

WORKOUT:

TUESDAY, 14

-
-
-
-

WORKOUT:

WEDNESDAY, 15

-
-
-
-

WORKOUT:

THURSDAY, 16

-
-
-
-

WORKOUT:

WORKOUT:

FRIDAY, 17

WORKOUT:

SATURDAY, 18

WORKOUT:

SUNDAY, 19

Weekly Eats:

To Do:

December 2021

MONDAY, 20

-
-
-
-

WORKOUT:

TUESDAY, 21

-
-
-
-

WORKOUT:

WEDNESDAY, 22

-
-
-
-

WORKOUT:

THURSDAY, 23

-
-
-
-

WORKOUT:

HAPPY + HEALTHY INTENTION:

....

WORKOUT:

....

....

FRIDAY, 24

WORKOUT:

....

SATURDAY, 25

WORKOUT:

....

SUNDAY, 26

Weekly Eats:

To Do:

December 2021

MONDAY, 27

-
-
-
-

WORKOUT:

TUESDAY, 28

-
-
-
-

WORKOUT:

WEDNESDAY, 29

-
-
-
-

WORKOUT:

THURSDAY, 30

-
-
-
-

WORKOUT:

....

WORKOUT:

....

....

....

FRIDAY, 31

....

....

....

WORKOUT:

....

....

....

SATURDAY, 1

....

....

....

WORKOUT:

....

....

....

SUNDAY, 2

....

....

....

Weekly Eats:

....

....

....

....

To Do:

....

....

....

....

....

Notes:

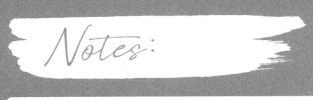
Notes:

CPSIA information can be obtained
at www.ICGtesting.com
Printed in the USA
LVHW020002140121
676450LV00016B/547